Pediatric Laboratory Interpretation

A Guide for the Pediatric Nurse

LOUISE D. JAKUBIK

Louise D. Jakubik, PhD, RN-BC
President and Chief Learning Officer
Nurse Builders
Philadelphia, PA

First Edition

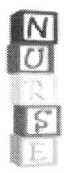

Nurse Builders, Philadelphia, PA

Pediatric Laboratory Interpretation

A Guide for the Pediatric Nurse

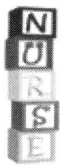

Louise D. Jakubik

Published by:
Nurse Builders
7715 Crittenden Street, Box 350
Philadelphia, PA 19118
www.nursebuilders.net

All rights reserved. No part of this book may be reproduced or transmitted in any form or by any means, electronic or mechanical, including photocopying, recording or by any information storage or retrieval system without written permission from the author, except for inclusion of brief quotations in a review.

Copyright © 2011 by Louise D. Jakubik.
First edition.
Printed in the United States of America.

Dedication

This book is dedicated to pediatric nurses who care for our children every day. Thank you for what you do. You are my heroes. You are the reason I do what I do every day to support you and promote you in your clinical practice.

About the Author

Louise Jakubik is the President and Chief Learning Officer in Nurse Builders, a nursing education firm that specializes in developing nurses and nursing organizations through continuing education, certification review, and organizational consultation. Dr. Jakubik received her BSN and MSN in acute and chronic nursing of children from University of Pennsylvania, and her PhD in nursing from Widener University. Her research agenda focuses on mentoring benefits for nurses and the organizations in which they work. Dr. Jakubik is a pediatric nursing expert whose professional life has been dedicated to building and developing nurses in clinical practice and leadership. She has held roles in pediatric nursing including staff nurse, pediatric nurse practitioner, clinical nurse specialist and nurse entrepreneur. She is a frequent national speaker on a variety of leadership and clinical topics including pediatric laboratory interpretation, certification review, mentoring, career development, and innovation in nursing education.

CONTENTS

Overview ... 7

1: Introduction to Pediatric Laboratory Interpretation ... 11

2: Pediatric Complete Blood Count (CBC) with Differential ... 15

3: Absolute Neutrophil Count (ANC) Calculation ... 47

4: Pediatric Fluid and Electrolytes and Dehydration ... 57

5: Pediatric Liver Function Tests (LFTs) ... 81

6: Pediatric Acid-Base Balance ... 103

References ... 113

Overview

Welcome to **Pediatric Laboratory Interpretation: A Guide for the Pediatric Nurse.** This book is intended as a practical guide to assist pediatric nurses in developing their knowledge and skills for pediatric laboratory interpretation. It is intended not only to expand your knowledge and thinking about pediatric laboratory interpretation, but also to assist you at the bedside as you interpret laboratory values for the children you care for.

This book is part of the Nurse Builders CE Series designed to develop the knowledge and skills of pediatric nurses. Additional teaching-learning tools for pediatric laboratory interpretation knowledge and skills development are also available such as laboratory values cards, audio CDs and video DVDs.

For more information about seminars and resources for pediatric laboratory interpretation, go to www.nursebuilders.net.

How to Use this Book

Pediatric laboratory interpretation can be a challenge. Most nurses receive inadequate information about how to interpret pediatric laboratory values in both their formal academic education and in their orientation and continuing education as clinical nurses. This book is designed to provide a practical approach to interpreting laboratory values commonly seen in clinical pediatric nursing. This step-by-step guide presents normal pediatric laboratory values as well as the implications for deviations from normal.

Warning – Disclaimer

This book is designed to provide you with information that will help you to interpret pediatric laboratory tests. Every effort has been made to make this book as accurate as possible.

10 | Pediatric Laboratory Interpretation

Chapter 1:
Introduction to Pediatric Laboratory Interpretation

Pediatric laboratory interpretation is a crucial component of a comprehensive assessment of the pediatric patient. However, many nurses find that their academic and clinical education do not adequately prepare them to interpret pediatric laboratory values as part of their clinical assessment of the pediatric patient. This handy little book will help to expand your knowledge regarding pediatric laboratory interpretation by examining each of the common pediatric laboratory tests, providing the normal pediatric laboratory parameters for each, and discussing the clinical implication for deviations from normal.

It is useful to think of the clinical assessment of a child as having three essential components: (1.) child and family history; (2.) pediatric physical assessment; and (3.) pediatric laboratory interpretation. Each of these components is important on its own, but together they give the healthcare provider a comprehensive, three-dimensional view of the child's health status.

In the following chapters, we will explore each of the common pediatric laboratory tests used in the care of pediatric patients. We will first explore the meaning and clinical indication of each laboratory parameter, including the normal laboratory values range for each laboratory test. Then, we will discuss the clinical implications for increases and decreases in each laboratory value. In each section, we will examine clinical case scenarios to apply the information we've learned.

Chapter 2:
Pediatric Complete Blood Count (CBC) with Differential

16 | *Pediatric Laboratory Interpretation*

Pediatric Complete Blood Count (CBC) and Differential

The CBC is one of the best and most commonly used pediatric laboratory tests. It is a single test which gives a terrific view of the child's overall health. It's a test used in primary care as a general health assessment and one that is also one of the most commonly used laboratory tests used for acutely ill children to assess their clinical status.

As a pediatric nurse it is important to know the components of the CBC and to understand their clinical implications.

In this chapter we will discuss the following information about the CBC and differential and their clinical implications:
- Blood and the formation of the cellular elements
- Documentation of the CBC, reticulocyte count, and differential
- Each cellular element in the standard CBC
- White blood cell (WBC) differential

- Implications of fluid status on CBC values

Blood
Blood has two components: (1.) plasma and (2.) formed elements. The *plasma* is the fluid component that is ninety percent water and ten percent solutes which include electrolytes and proteins. The *formed elements* are the cellular components such as the white blood cells, red blood cells, and platelets.

Hematopoiesis
Hematopoiesis is the formation of blood. The *hematopoetic stem cell* is the origin of all blood cells. Hematopoetic organs are the bone marrow (myeloid tissue) and the lymphatic system. The bone marrow, located in long bones, ribs, sternum, vertebrae, is the primary site of blood cell formation. *T Lymphocytes* are also formed in the bone marrow and then migrate to the lymphatic system for maturation. The lymphatic system, comprised of the lymph nodes, spleen, thymus, and tonsils is a particularly important site of hematopoiesis for the young fetus together with the liver and bone marrow.

FORMED ELEMENTS:

Let's first take a look at the formed elements in the CBC. These are the traditional values that we examine when looking at the typical CBC. Later, we'll talk about the impact that the plasma has on these formed elements.

Documentation of the CBC

One of the first challenges of a clinical nurse is to be able to accurately gather the CBC values from the pediatric patient's medical record. The ability to gather this data depends on the nurse's ability to understand basic documentation principles in the medical record. The standard way to document a CBC in the medical record is shown on the next page. The white blood cell (WBC) is written to the left; the hemoglobin (Hgb) is placed on top; the hematocrit (Hct) is placed on the bottom; and the platelet (Plt) count is placed to the right. If a reticulocyte count, a separate test, is reported then it is written out to the right as shown. The WBC differential, a separate test, is written out as shown.

$$\text{WBC} > \genfrac{}{}{0pt}{}{\text{Hgb}}{\text{Hct}} < \text{Plt}$$

Retic = ____

Bands =
Segs =
Lymphs =
Monos =
Eos =
Basos =

Let's take a look at each of these cellular components of the CBC. We'll describe each component and its clinical implication as well as the meaning of deviations from normal. At the end of this chapter, we'll examine case studies to apply this information to clinical practice.

A word about deviations from normal
As you are considering each of the cellular elements and their deviations from normal, it is helpful to think about the bone marrow, where each cellular element is made, as being on a dining room dimmer switch. Normally a dining room dimmer switch is on a sliding lever or a dial. In either case, the lever or dial

is placed in the middle for fairly moderate lighting as you'd use to eat a meal at dinner time. However, if you want to set the mood for a romantic or formal dinner, you can slide down the lever or turn down the dial so that the lighting is very dim. One can even turn it off in this manner. However, if the atmosphere calls for very bright lighting, you can turn the lever or dial all of the way up so it is a very bright and stimulating environment. The bone marrow works exactly like this. Normally, the bone marrow is producing at a moderate rate, just as if the dining room dimmer switch were placed right in the middle (not too bright and not too dim). Certain conditions or clinical situations will cause the bone marrow to be suppressed. Think of bone marrow suppression as having the dining room dimmer switch turned down. At other times, the bone marrow will be stimulated to over-produce. In these cases, you should think of the dining room dimmer switch as being turned up. Each time you consider a patient's diagnosis and interpret the patient's CBC, think about the bone marrow as the dining room dimmer switch and whether or not it is being turned up, turned down, or is unaffected.

White Blood Cell (WBC, Leukocyte)
The white blood cell is the cellular element whose primary job is to fight infection and attack foreign material. The range is 4,500 – 17,000 mm^3 which is typically abbreviated at 1/1000 of the actual value as follows: 4.5 – 17. The lifespan of the WBC is hours to days.

Clinical Implications
The clinical implications for an increased WBC count are infection, tissue necrosis, bone marrow malignancies, and inflammation. The most common cause of an increase in the WBC count is infection. Bone marrow malignancies, however, can also cause an increase in the WBC because they disrupt the bone marrow and may cause inappropriate release of WBCs.

The clinical implications for a decreased WBC count are infections and conditions or medications that suppress or weaken the immune system or exhaust the bone marrow. Infection is typically considered as a cause of an increase in the WBC count, but severe infection or sepsis can overwhelm the immune system causing a decrease in the WBC count. This is particularly true among neonates who have a decreased immune system function and are, therefore, at risk for a decreased rather than increased WBC as the result of an infection.

WBC Differential

The WBC differential is a laboratory test that breaks down the overall WBC count into the six different types of white blood cells that are contained within the overall WBC count. Each type is expressed as a percentage (%) of the total WBC count. Therefore, the sum of the components of the WBC differential must add up to 100%. So naturally as one component goes up, the other components will go down.

The WBC differential is the *informative* component of the WBC because each different type of WBC contained within the WBC differential responds to different types of infections. A rise in a particular type of WBC, therefore, can indicate the type of infection that the child may have. The WBC differential is frequently used as an initial test to give clinicians clues about the patient's condition that may be used to guide clinical management of the patient prior to other clinical results such as blood and other cultures.

The components of the WBC differential are:
- Neutrophils
    - Band neutrophils (called "bands")
    - Segmented neutrophils (called "segs")
- Lymphocytes
- Monocytes
- Eosinophils
- Basophils

Neutrophils (31-57%)
The neutrophils are the first line of defense against infection. They are broken down into two types: (1.) bands or stabs (hereafter called bands) and (2.) segs. The bands, whose normal value is zero (0) are the immature neutrophils that are not normally present in the systemic circulation. While the segs, whose normal value is 31% - 57%, are the mature neutrophils that are released into the systemic circulation to fight infection.

Clinical Implications
The clinical implications for <u>increased neutrophils</u> (neutrophilia) include: bacterial infection, some inflammatory conditions, tissue damage, and malignancies of the bone marrow (leukemia). A rise in neutrophils in general is

consistent with a *bacterial Infection*. A rise in *bands* in particular is highly suggestive of *bacterial infection*.

Clinical implications for <u>decreased neutrophils</u> (neutropenia) include: some viral conditions, overwhelming infection that exhausts the bone marrow, cancer treatment drugs, certain antibiotics and psychotropic drugs, and some hereditary disorders. Newborns with sepsis are at higher risk for developing neutropenia because of their immature immune systems.

Monocytes (4-7%)
Monocytes are the second line of defense against infection. They typically indicate a *viral infection*.

Clinical Implications
Clinical implications for <u>increased monocytes</u> (monocytosis) include: monocytic leukemia, ulcerative colitis, viral diseases such as mononucleosis and herpes zoster, parasitic diseases such as Rocky Mountain Spotted Fever. In general though, an <u>increased monocyte</u> count is associated with *viral infection*.

Clinical implications for a decreased monocytes count (monopenia) includes: some forms of leukemia and bone marrow failure or suppression.

Lymphocytes (35-61%)
The lymphocytes, produced in the lymphatic system, are broken down into the B lymphocytes (B cells) and the T lymphocytes (T cells). The B cells are responsible for humoral immunity, while the T cells are responsible for cell-mediated immunity. An increase in the overall lymphocyte count (lymphocytosis) indicates a *viral infection*.

Clinical Implications
Clinical implications for increased lymphocytes (lymphocytosis) include: viral infections (most common), *bacterial* or *allergic conditions* (less common).

Clinical implications for decreased lymphocytes (lymphopenia) include: corticosteroid therapy, adrenocortical hyperfunction, stress, and shock.

Helpful Hint: Remember, when one component of the WBC differential goes up, other components will necessarily go down. Therefore, one can see monopenia and/or lymphopenia in the face of other, non-viral infections.

Eosinophils (2-4%)
The eosinophils are released in response to *allergic disorders* and *parasitic infections*.

Clinical Implications
Clinical implications for increased eosinophils (eosinophilia) include: asthma, hay fever, and drug reactions.

Clinical implications for decreased eosinophils (eosinopenia) include: corticosteroid therapy, adrenocortical hyperfunction, stress, and shock.

Basophils (0-1%)
The basophils are responsible for histamine release and are released in response to inflammatory states such as a *systemic allergic reaction*.

Clinical Implications
Clinical implications for <u>increased basophils</u> (basophilia) include: chronic inflammatory and hypersensitivity reactions.

Clinical implications for <u>decreased basophils</u> (basopenia) include: corticosteroid therapy, adrenocortical hyperfunction, stress, and shock.

Shifts

So what is all of the buzz about *shifts*? The bottom line is that *shifts* are slang terms that clinicians use to describe the direction of the WBC count to the bacterial or the viral end. While these are slang terms, clinicians use them all of the time. So if you don't know what they mean it makes it hard to communicate. I will never forget my first experience as a pediatric nurse communicating about *shifts*. I was a young pediatric nurse with about a year of clinical experience. I was at that point in my career where I was just moving out of the novice phase, where I'd started to gain some confidence and to feel like I knew a bit more than I didn't. I was working night shift and received report over the phone from the emergency department (ED) nurse about a young baby who was coming in with a fever. The ED nurse gave me a full report on the patient and at the end said, "Oh and she has a *left shift,*" and then hung up the phone. Immediately, I felt stupid. I had no idea what a *left shift* was. So I did what many new nurses do, which is to do nothing and tell no one. I always regret that I had not taken that as a teachable moment to find out in that moment what a *left shift* was. A few years later, I was a pediatric nurse practitioner in hematology and began my journey to explore pediatric laboratory interpretation and to share the information with every nurse who would listen. My point in this story is that while *left and right shifts* are slang, if people talk in slang about a patient's condition, we as clinical nurses need to know what that slang means.

So what's a *left shift*?
A *left shift* is specifically an *increase in bands*. A *left shift* indicates a *bacterial infection*. Bands that are released into the systemic circulation indicate that the bone marrow is responding to bacterial infection by releasing these immature neutrophils to fight the infection.

The origin of the *left shift* comes from when the laboratory wrote the WBC differential from left to right on the paper as follows: bands, segs, monos, lymphs, eos, and basos. Since the bands were furthest to the left, this became known as a *left shift*. While technically, a *left shift* is considered an *increase in the bands*, in practice many clinicians consider it an *increase in the combined bands and segs*.

***Memory Jogger:** One way to remember that bands are consistent with a bacterial infection is to remember that bands and bacterial both start with "ba."*

So what's a *right shift*?
Technically, there is no such thing as a *right shift*. In practice, if someone refers to a *right shift* they are referring to a *rise in the monocytes and lymphocytes*. A *right shift* indicates a *viral infection*. This is the reason that we don't typically refer to right shifts. Viral infections, while common, are not typically what we are looking to discover and treat in an acute pediatric patient environment. Viruses are typically not as exciting for the clinician and also require less intervention. Hence, there is often a lack of clinical reference to a *right shift*.

Red Blood Cell (RBC, Erythrocyte)
The RBC transports oxygenated hemoglobin (Hgb) to the tissues of the body and plays a small role in the maintenance of acid-base equilibrium. The lifespan of the RBC is 120 days.

Production of RBCs is regulated by 2 things: (1.) tissue oxygenation and (2.) renal production of erythropoietin. Tissue hypoxia stimulates the kidneys to produce erythropoietin, which then stimulates the bone marrow to release RBC's. **It is the ability of the RBCs to transport oxygen to the tissues of the body that regulates the production of RBCs not the number of RBC's circulating.** What this means is that the bone marrow makes more RBCs when the body has increased needs for oxygen carrying capacity.

Clinical Implications
Clinical implications for increased RBCs (polycythemia) include: congenital heart disease, chronic hypoxia, high altitudes, and polycythemia vera.

Clinical implications for decreased RBCs include: renal disease, hematological conditions involving RBC destruction, iron deficiency, vitamin B12 deficiency, blood loss/hemorrhage, and bone marrow suppression.

RBC Indices

The RBC Indices measure the size and Hgb content of the RBC. They are calculated based on mathematical formulas that reflect the relationships among the RBC, Hgb, and hematocrit (Hct). The RBC Indices are primarily used to differentiate between different types of anemia.

Helpful Hint: Look first at the Hgb to determine if the child is anemic (low hemoglobin). If the child has anemia, then look at the RBC Indices to determine if the RBC is normal. Typically, abnormalities in the RBC indices give us clues about the source of the anemia.

The RBC Indices include the following: mean corpuscular volume (MCV); mean corpuscular hemoglobin (MCH); mean corpuscular hemoglobin concentration (MCHC); and red cell distribution width (RDW). Let's take a moment and examine each of these.

Pediatric Laboratory Interpretation | 33

Mean Corpuscular Volume (MCV)

The MCV indicates the average size of the RBC. The MCV is described as either normocytic (normal cell size), macrocytic (large cell size), or microcytic (small cell size). Let's take a look at each one.

Clinical Implications

Normocytic RBCs are a normal size with a value of 75-94 femtolitres (fl) with some variation based on age and gender.

Macrocytic RBCs are large in size with a value greater than 94 fl. Clinical implications for an increased MCV include: folate or vitamin B12 deficiency, aplastic anemia, and immune hemolytic anemia.

Microcytic RBCs are small in size with a value of less than 75 fl. Clinical implications for a decreased MCV include: iron deficiency anemia, lead poisoning, and thalassemia.

Mean Corpuscular Hemoglobin (MCH)

The MCH measures the average weight of Hgb per RBC with a normal range of 25-33 picrograms (pg).

Clinical Implications
Clinical implications for an increased MCH are the same as for the MCV which include: folate or vitamin B12 deficiency, aplastic anemia, and immune hemolytic anemia.

Clinical implications for a decreased MCH are the same as for the MCV which include: iron deficiency anemia, lead poisoning, and thalassemia.

Mean Corpuscular Hemoglobin Concentration (MCHC)
The MCHC measures the average concentration of Hgb per RBC and is described in three ways: normochromic, hyperchromic, and hypochromic.

Clinical Implications
Normochromic RBCs contain a normal Hgb concentration with a value of 33-36%.

Hyperchromic RBCs contain an increased concentration of Hgb per RBC with a value of greater than 36%. Clinical implications for increased MCHC include: hereditary spherocytosis. Interestingly, this is the only clinical diagnosis which is consistent with an increased MCHC and, therefore, is a component of the diagnostic evaluation for this diagnosis.

Hypochromic RBCs contain a decreased concentration of Hgb per RBC with a value of less than 33%. Clinical implications for decreased MCHC increased iron deficiency and thalassemia.

Red Cell Distribution Width (RDW)
The RDW measures the uniformity of RBC size with a normal range of 11.5 – 14.5.

Clinical Implications
An increased RDW is called *anisocytosis* and indicates greater cell size variability. Clinical implications for increased RDW include: iron deficiency anemia, folic acid deficiency anemia, and vitamin B12 deficiency anemia.

Reticulocyte/"Retic" Count (0.5% - 1.5%)
The reticulocyte count, often called "retic," is an immature RBC. The normal retic range is 0.5%-1.5% and indicates active RBC production from the bone marrow. It is used as an indirect measure of hematopoiesis.

Clinical Implications
Clinical implications for <u>increased reticulocytes</u> (reticulocytosis) include: acute anemia and chronic hemolytic anemia (sickle cell disease, hereditary spherocytosis).

Clinical implications for <u>decreased reticulocytes</u> (reticulocytopenia) include: bone marrow failure syndrome, infectious bone marrow suppression, iron deficiency anemia, vitamin B12 deficiency anemia, and folate deficiency anemia.

Helpful Hint: The retic and the hemoglobin (Hgb or Hb) are <u>inversely related</u>, which means that as the Hgb goes down, the retic goes up. When the Hgb is normal (11.5 -14.5), the retic is normal (0.5% - 1.5%). As the Hgb goes down, the retic should necessarily increase which indicates that the bone barrow is responding by <u>turning up the dining room dimer switch</u>. This natural response of the bone marrow to produce more immature RBCs (reticulocytes) in the face of a falling or low baseline Hgb is the normal feedback loop upon which RBCs are made.

Hemoglobin (Hgb or Hb)

Hgb is the component of the RBC that binds oxygen and delivers it to the tissues of the body. The normal range for a pediatric Hgb is 11.5 – 14.5 g/dl with some variation based on age and gender. There are various types of Hgb that are produced depending upon the stage in life and any abnormalities in the genes which regulate hemoglobin. The two basic types of normal hemoglobin are: fetal hemoglobin (Hgb F) and adult hemoglobin (Hgb A). Each type of Hgb is composed of four (4) globin chains which determine its type. Hgb F contains two (2) alpha and two (2) gamma chains. Hgb A contains two (2) alpha and two (2) beta chains.

Clinical Implications

Clinical implications for <u>increased hemoglobin</u> include: congenital heart disease, chronic hypoxia, high altitudes, polycythemia vera, and fluid loss (dehydration).

Clinical implications for <u>decreased hemoglobin</u> (anemia) can be categorized into four (4) causes:
1. Decreased Production: aplastic anemia, renal disease, iron deficiency, bone marrow suppression

2. Increased Destruction: sickle cell disease, hereditary spherocytosis
3. Blood Loss: hemorrhage
4. Other: fluid volume overload

Hematocrit (Hct)
The Hct reflects the percentage of packed RBC to whole blood. The relationship between Hct and Hgb is a fixed relationship of three (3) times the Hgb value. Therefore, the Hct rises and falls in the same direction and for the same clinical reasons as does Hgb.

Clinical Implications
Clinical implications for an increased hematocrit (same as for Hgb) include: more cells or less fluid. Clinical diagnoses which cause an increase in the Hgb concentration such as *tetralogy of fallot* will cause an increase in Hct. In this condition, the bone marrow is stimulated to make more RBCs containing Hgb because the child is chronically hypoxic. *Dehydration* will cause an increase in the Hgb concentration and therefore will *falsely increase* the Hgb and Hct. Correction of dehydration will lower the Hgb and Hct to their true values.

Pediatric Laboratory Interpretation | 39

Helpful Hint: Whenever you rehydrate a dehydrated child, the Hgb and Hct will <u>decrease</u>. If a child is brought to your emergency department with fever, dehydration, and a Hgb of 6, and then receives two (2) 20ml/kg IV fluid boluses of 0.9% normal saline, his Hgb <u>will go down</u> after the child receives the fluid resuscitation described above.

Clinical implications for <u>decreased hematocrit</u> (same as for Hgb) include: fewer cells or more fluid. Clinical diagnoses which are consistent with RBC hemolysis (breakdown) such as *sickle cell disease* will cause a decrease in Hct. In this condition, RBCs' lifespan are only 20 days and therefore hemolyze much more quickly than normal RBCs, which live for 120 days. The fast rate of RBC hemolysis in this condition causes a <u>decreased baseline Hgb and Hct</u> thereby decreasing the concentration of cells per unit volume. *Overhydration* will cause a decrease in the Hgb concentration and with therefore *falsely decrease* the Hgb and Hct. Correcting the overhydration will increase the Hgb and Hct to their true values.

Platelet (Plt)

Platelets are the cellular components needed to form a clot. The normal range is 150,000 – 450,000/mm³ which is generally abbreviated as 150-450 or 1/1000 of the actual value. The platelets are regulated by thrombopoietin but their mechanism of action is largely unknown.

Clinical Implications

Clinical implications for increased platelets (thrombocytosis) include: acute blood loss, myeloproliferative disease, and polycythemia vera.

Clinical implications for decreased platelets (thrombocytopenia) include three (3) main causes:
1. Decreased Production: leukemias, other primary bone marrow failure syndromes
2. Increased Destruction: idiopathic thrombocytopenia purpura (ITP), certain drugs
3. Abnormal Pooling: splenic sequestration, splenomegaly

Case Studies

1. Brian is a 6 year old who is admitted to your inpatient unit after coming to your emergency department with a fever and the following CBC results:

    $$\begin{array}{c} 12.8 \\ 25 >\text{----------}< 222 \\ 37 \end{array} \quad \text{Retic} = 1.2$$

    Bands = 4   Segs = 60   Lymphs = 28
    Monos = 4   Eos = 3   Basos = 1

    a. What values in the CBC are abnormal?

    b. Is this a left or a right shift?

    c. What does the shift indicate?

2. Brooke is a 10 year old who comes to your emergency department with a complaint of pain and the following CBC results:

$$15> \frac{7}{22} <324$$

Retic = 16

a. What values in the CBC are abnormal?

b. What do these CBC abnormalities indicate?

3. Peter is a 13 month old infant who comes to your primary care clinic with a complaint of malaise and the following CBC results:

$$\begin{array}{c} 8 \\ 10> \text{-----------} <286 \\ 25 \qquad \text{Retic} = 1.0 \end{array}$$

RDW = 17   MCV = 69
MCH = 22   MCHC = 30

a. What values in the CBC are abnormal?

b. What do these CBC abnormalities indicate?

c. Name one diagnosis that could explain these laboratory values.

Answers

Case Study #1
    a. The white blood cells, bands, and segs are elevated.

    b. This represents a left shift since the elevation is in the bands in particular and the bands and segs in general.

    c. A left shift indicates a bacterial infection.

Case Study #2
    a. Brooke's hemoglobin and hematocrit are low and her retic count is elevated.

    b. These CBC values indicate that Brooke is anemic and her bone marrow is responding by *over-producing* in order to compensate for the low hemoglobin. This is indicative of conditions like sickle cell disease.

Case Study #3
   a. The following values are low: Hgb, MCV, MCH, and MCHC. The RDW is elevated which indicates *anisocytosis*.

   b. Peter is anemic with abnormalities in his RBCs which show an increased cell size variability, a low concentration and weight of Hgb per RBC, and a small RBC size.

   c. Iron deficiency anemia

Chapter 3:
Absolute Neutrophil Count (ANC) Calculation

Absolute Neutrophil Count (ANC)

The absolute neutrophil count (ANC) represents the actual number rather than the percentage of neutrophils contained within the WBC differential. Recall that the neutrophils are the bands and the segs and that they are each expressed as a percentage of the overall WBC count. To obtain the ANC it is necessary to perform a calculation that takes the percentage of bands and segs and turns them into a true number rather than a percentage. This ANC value is important because it indicates the decree of immune system function integrity.

Normal Range (> 1000)
The normal range for an ANC is greater than 1000. However, most children's ANC is far higher than that.

Neutropenia (ANC < 1000)
Neutropenia is defined as an ANC of less than 1000. An ANC count of 500 – 1000 indicates a moderate risk for infection, while an ANC count of less than 500 indicates a severe risk of life-threatening infection. There are a variety of causes of neutropenia including:

chemotherapy, immunosupression (steroid therapy), chronic benign neutropenia of childhood, and syndromes affecting the immune system.

Calculation
There are three (3) calculation methods to calculate the ANC as listed below:
- Method #1: (Bands + Segs)% X true WBC = ANC

- Method #2: {(Bands + Segs) X WBC} / 100 = ANC

- Method #3: (Bands + Segs) X (Abbreviated WBC X 10) = ANC

Example:
A child's CBC is the following:
WBC = 10,000   Hgb = 13   Hct = 39   Plt = 398
Bands = 0   Segs = 56   Mon = 7   Lymphs = 34
Eos = 2   Basos = 1
- Method #1: (0 + 56)% X 10,000 = 5,600

- Method #2: 56 X 10,000 = 560,000/100 = 5,600

- Method #3: 56 X (10 X 10 = 100) = 5,600

Helpful Hint: If the WBC count is normal (5-17.5) then the ANC will be normal. A helpful rule is to remember the number "5" (the fingers on one hand). If the WBC is 5 or less, then calculate the ANC. Otherwise, it is safe to assume that the ANC is normal.

Case Studies

1. You are taking care of a 3 year old hospitalized for an immune deficiency. His CBC is the following:

   $$\begin{array}{c} 12 \\ 4 >\text{----------}< 187 \\ 36 \end{array}$$

   Bands = 0   Segs = 20   Lymphs = 65
   Monos = 9   Eos = 4   Basos = 2

   a. What is his ANC?

   b. What does it indicate?

2. You are a nurse working in the pediatric emergency room. You receive the following CBC results for one of your patients:

$$\begin{array}{c} 13 \\ 12 > \text{-----------} < 256 \\ 38 \end{array}$$

Bands = 0   Segs = 53   Lymphs = 40
Mons = 4   Eos = 3   Basos = 0

a. What is the child's ANC?

b. What does it indicate?

Answers

Case Study #1
a. ANC = 800
   Method #1: $(0 + 20)\% \times 4{,}000 = 800$
   Method #2: $(0 + 20) \times 4{,}000 / 100 = 800$
   Method #3: $(0 + 20) \times (4 \times 10 = 40) = 800$

b. Neutropenia

Case Study #2
a. ANC = 6360
   Method #1: $(0 + 53)\% \times 12{,}000 = 6360$
   Method #2: $(0 + 53) \times 12{,}000 / 100 = 6360$
   Method #3: $(0 + 53) \times (12 \times 10 = 120) = 6360$

b. intact immune system

Chapter 4:
Pediatric Fluid and Electrolytes and Dehydration

Pediatric Fluid and Electrolytes and Dehydration

Children are at particular risk for fluid and electrolyte imbalances and dehydration. Therefore, it is important that pediatric nurses understand how to interpret pediatric electrolytes and how to assess pediatric hydration status.

In this chapter we will discuss the following information about pediatric fluid and electrolytes and dehydration:
- Normal pediatric fluid distribution
- Pediatric hydration assessment
- Maintenance fluid calculation
- Pediatric dehydration assessment and classification
- Treatment options for pediatric dehydration

Normal Pediatric Fluid Distribution
The following are key difference in the fluid distribution among children as compared to adults:
1. Higher proportion of body water accounts for their weight
2. Greater proportion of body water is in the ECF compartment
3. Greater proportional body surface area
4. Higher metabolic rate
5. Immature kidneys and immature homeostatic regulation (buffer) system
6. Increased insensible water losses
7. Decreased ability to regulate temperature (among young infants) through sweating or shivering

Total Body Water: Distribution by Fluid Compartment
Fluid is contained within two (2) major compartments in the body: (1.) intracellular (inside the cell) and (2.) extracellular (outside the cell). The extracellular fluid is then further divided into the intravascular (inside the vessel) and extravascular (outside the vessel) spaces.

The intracellular fluid (ICF) is contained inside the cell. It is the larger fluid compartment with potassium (K^+) as the main electrolyte. The extracellular fluid (ECF) is outside the cell. It is the smaller fluid compartment with sodium (Na) as the main electrolyte. The intravascular fluid is the ECF that is inside the vessel (plasma) and the extravascular fluid is the ECF that is outside the vessel which includes: interstitial fluid (pulmonary) and transcellular fluid (cerebrospinal fluid).

How and why does fluid move between the fluid compartments?
There are four (4) mechanisms which facilitate the movement of fluid between compartments including:
 1. Osmosis
 2. Facilitated Diffusion
 3. Active Transport
 4. Filtration

Osmolality
Osmosis is the number of particles (proteins and electrolytes) per liter of water. Sodium (Na) is the major intravascular cation. Normally, the osmolality between the fluid

compartments is approximately equal so there is movement of fluid between compartments.

Osmosis

Osmosis is the movement of water through a semi-permiable membrane from a compartment with high water potential (low solute concentration) to a compartment with low water potential (high solute concentration). Water moves in order to equalize the solute concentration on both sides of the membrane. More specifically, water moves from a less-concentrated (hypotonic) solution to a more-concentrated (hypertonic) solution.

Osmotic Pressure

Osmotic pressure is the force necessary to prevent osmosis. Osmotic pressure increases as the solute concentration of a solution increases. Free water moves from an area of LOW osmolality to and area of HIGH osmolality.

Tonicity

Tonicity refers to the strength of a solution. *Isotonic solutions* have the same osmolality as plasma. Because there is no solute concentration difference between compartments, isotonic solutions have no effect on cells because they do not stimulate movement of water into or out of the cells. *Hypotonic solutions* have a lower solute concentration and lower plasma oncotic pressure as compared to plasma. *Hypotonic solutions*, therefore, cause RBCs to swell and burst (hemolysis) because they cause water to rush into the cells. *Hypertonic solutions* have a higher solute concentration and higher plasma oncotic pressure as compared to plasma. *Hypertonic solutions*, therefore, cause RBCs to shrink (crenate) due to the movement of water out of the cell.

Pediatric Hydration Assessment Components
- Level of Consciousness
- Vital Signs
- Mucous Membranes
- Skin Turgor
- Skin Color
- Urine output and Specific Gravity
- Tear Output
- Capillary Refill
- Pulses
- Fontanel
- Eyes

Assessment of Intake and Output
Assessment of Output
- Urine volume
    - Minimum of 1cc/kg/hr
    - Normal of 2-4cc/kg/hr
- Daily weights
- Stool output
    - Frequency, consistency, color, pain

Assessment of Intake:
Pediatric Maintenance Fluid Requirements

Pediatric maintenance fluid requirements are the water and electrolytes required to sustain the expenditure of normal physiologic activities. Pediatric maintenance fluid requirements provide a baseline for determining the amount of fluid a child requires based on weight. This calculation does not take into consideration clinical conditions which might affect the child's needs for more or less fluid. Adjustments to individual fluid requirements should be made based on the child's particular clinical condition.

Conditions that are associated with <u>increased</u> pediatric maintenance fluid requirements include: fever, diarrhea, vomiting, burns, shock, and sickle cell disease. Conditions that are associated with <u>decreased</u> pediatric maintenance fluid requirements include: renal failure/disease, congestive heart failure, and post-operative care.

The standard method for calculating the pediatric maintenance fluid requirement is by using either the short or long version of the Holiday-Segar maintenance fluid calculation formula. It is important to note that these formulas are not intended to be used in pre-term infants or in full term infants younger than 2 week of age.

Maintenance Fluid Calculation:

	Short Version (hourly)	
Weight (kg)	X ___ ml/hour	
1st 10 kg (0-10 kg)	4 ml/hour	a
2nd 10 kg (11-20 kg)	2 ml/hour	b
Kg > 20 kg	1 ml/hour	c
	a + b + c = **X ml/hour**	

	Long Version (daily)	
Weight (kg)	X ___ ml/day	
1st 10 kg (0-10 kg)	100 ml/day	a
2nd 10 kg (11-20 kg)	50 ml/day	b
Kg > 20 kg	20 ml/day	c
	a + b + c = **X ml/day**	

Pediatric Dehydration Assessment and Classification

- Dehydration - Definition
    - Fluid volume deficit
    - Total output > total intake

- Classification
    - Degree
    - Type

- Clinical Manifestations
    - Weight Loss
    - Specific Clinical Symptoms
        - Reflective of the degree of fluid depletion in the intravascular space
        - See Hydration Assessment Table

Hydration Assessment

Degree of Dehydration	Normal	Mild Dehydration	Moderate Dehydration	Severe Dehydration
Fluid Level	Normal	5% weight loss Or <50 ml/kg deficit	10% weight loss Or 50 - 90 ml/kg deficit	15% weight loss Or >100 ml/kg
Tear Formation	Big, wet tears	Present	Decreased to absent	Absent
Level of Consciousness	Developmentally appropriate	Alert and oriented; may be irritable	Irritability and/or decreased activity and/or confusion	Lethargic, drowsy, unconscious
Mucous Membrane	Normal	Normal to dry	Dry	Very dry, parched
Skin Elasticity/ Turgor	Normal	Normal	Slight delay in return	Notable delay in return
Urine Output	Normal	Normal (concentrated: increased specific gravity)	Decreased (oliguria) with increased specific gravity	Absent (anuria)
Fontanel (<18 months) and eyes	Normal	Normal to slightly sunken	Slightly sunken	Severely sunken
Heart Rate	Normal	Normal to slight tachycardia up to 10 bpm	Moderate tachycardia of 10 - 20 bpm	Extreme tachycardia (HR increase 20 bpm) to bradycardia
Respirations	Normal	Normal	Normal to tachypnic	Rate and pattern changes
Blood Pressure	Normal	Normal	Normal to mild hypotension	Severe hypotension

Hydration Assessment (Continued)

Degree of Dehydration	Normal	Mild Dehydration	Moderate Dehydration	Severe Dehydration
Pulses	Strong	Strong	Decreased peripheral pulses; difficult to locate	Weak to absent peripheral pulses
Neurovascular Assessment	Warm, pink skin Cap refill = brisk (< 2 sec)	Warm, pink skin Cap refill = brisk (< 2 sec)	Warm to cool skin Pink to pale Cap refill = slight delay	Cold Mottled, grey, cyanotic Cap refill = delayed (> 3 sec)
Treatment	N/A	Usually outpatient treatment Oral rehydration therapy (ORT) using an isotonic rehydration solution such as Pedialyte; typically administered rapidly over several hours	Inpatient treatment is common Rapid fluid resuscitation to restore intravascular volume (and systemic perfusion) using an IV fluid bolus (10 ml/kg) with an isotonic rehydrating solution such as Normal Saline. Then, IV + PO fluids to maintain and restore fluid deficits over 24 – 48 hours.	Treated for hypovolemic shock in the ER. Rapid fluid resuscitation to restore intravascular volume (and systemic perfusion) using an IV fluid bolus (10-20 ml/kg) with an isotonic rehydrating solution such as Normal Saline. Then, IV fluids to replace maintenance requirements plus 100+ml/kg fluid deficits over 24–48 hrs.

Degrees of Dehydration (i.e. Severity Level)

The degree of dehydration a child experiences is described based on the relative amount of fluid deficit contained in the ICF and ECF compartments as follows:

- Mild
  - Most common severity level of dehydration
  - 5% weight loss from pre-illness weight
  - <50 ml/kg fluid loss
  - Clinical manifestations (see table)
  - Treatment (see table)

- Moderate
  - 10% weight loss from pre-illness weight
  - 50 – 90 ml/kg fluid loss
  - Clinical manifestations (see table)
  - Treatment (see table)

- Severe
  - 15% weight loss from pre-illness weight
  - > 100 ml/kg fluid loss

- Clinical manifestations (see table)
- Treatment (see table)

Types of Dehydration (i.e. Classification by Sodium Level)

The type of dehydration is determined based on the degree of sodium (Na) and water losses and divided into three categories: isotonic (isonatremic), hypotonic (hyponatremic), and hypertonic (hypernatremic).

- **Isotonic (Isonatremic) Dehydratrion**

Isotonic dehydration is the most common type of dehydration (70% of cases of pediatric dehydration). In this type of dehydration, sodium and water losses occur in balanced proportions and as a result, the serum sodium (Na) is normal (130 – 150 mEq/L). There are no osmotic forces in this type of dehydration, meaning that the osmolality is equal between the ECF and ICF and, thus, there is no movement of fluid across the cell wall between the ECF and ICF compartments. In this type of dehydration, the fluid depletion is in the ECF with depletion primarily in the circulating blood volume within the intravascular space.

- **Hypotonic (Hyponatremic) Dehydration**

Hypotonic dehydration occurs in 10-15% of cases of pediatric dehydration. In this type of dehydration, the depletion of sodium is greater than the depletion of water and, therefore, the serum Na is less than 130 mEq/L. Water shifts from the ECF to the ICF because the Na is higher in the ICF. This movement of water helps to establish equilibrium of Na but *increases* the relative severity of the dehydration. The result is that the signs and symptoms of dehydration are typically more severe with smaller fluid losses and, therefore, there is an early onset of more severe clinical signs and symptoms of dehydration.

- **Hypertonic (Hypernatremic) Dehydration**

Hypertonic dehydration occurs in 10-15% of cases of pediatric dehydration. It is the most dangerous form of dehydration among children. In this type of dehydration, the depletion of water is greater than the depletion of Na and, therefore, the serum Na is greater than 150mEq/L. Water shifts from the ICF to the ECF because the Na is higher in the ECF. This movement of water helps to establish equilibrium of Na but masks the severity of dehydration as fluid moves into the ECF. Clinical signs and symptoms of dehydration, therefore, occur much later and require a greater severity of fluid loss in order to appear. Shock is less apparent until dehydration is very severe. Seizures and neurologic symptoms are most closely associated with this type of dehydration.

Interpretation of the Urine Specific Gravity and Basic Metabolic Panel (BMP)

Urine Specific Gravity

The urine specific gravity provides an assessment of the degree of urine concentration and can be an important initial sign of dehydration in children. Urine specific gravity is considered elevated if it is greater than 1.020. It is important to note that the kidneys do not concentrate urine normally as adult kidneys do until the child has reached two years of age. The urine specific gravity, therefore, is a useful clinical assessment parameter for dehydration in older children to identify concentrated urine, but is of limited use in assessing dehydration in children younger than 2 years.

Pediatric Laboratory Interpretation | 73

Basic Metabolic Panel (BMP)
<u>Sodium / Chloride/ BUN / Glucose
Potassium/ CO2 / Creatinine</u>

Sodium (Na+)

Hypotonic Dehydration	Isotonic Dehydration	Hypertonic Dehydration
130meq/L	130-150 meq/L	>150meq/L

Potassium (K+)
- Moves from ICF to ECF
- Kidney function is decreased during dehydration so normal K+ excretion does not occur
- Serum K+ levels can increase and then rapidly decrease during rehydration

Chloride (Cl-)
- Component of hydrochloric acid located in stomach
- Serum levels decrease in dehydration
- Key component in determining etiology and in maintaining acid-base balance

Acid-Base Imbalance
- Metabolic Acidosis
  - Net loss of bicarbonate (HCO3-)
  - Increase in acids
  - pH of <7.35
- Metabolic Alkalosis
  - Increase in bicarbonate (HCO3-)
  - Loss of acids
  - pH of >7.45

BMP in the child who is "dry"
- BUN increases, but Creatinine remains within normal limits
- BUN to Creatinine ratio is ~ 10 to 1
- If ratio is $\geq$ 20/1, renal failure may occur

BMP in child who is dehydrated with renal involvement
- BUN and Creatinine increase
- Dehydration can lead to renal failure so watch for increasing Creatinine

BMP in child with severe vomiting
- Decreased Sodium
- Decreased Potassium
- Decreased Chloride
- Increased Bicarbonate (HCO3-)
- Increased CO2

BMP in child with diarrhea
- Sodium can be increased, decreased, or remain within normal limits
- Decreased Bicarbonate (lost in stool)
- Increased BUN

Treatment

Rehydration Points to Remember
- Oral is better if child is well enough to attempt oral intake.
- IV Fluids should be free of potassium (K) until after the child has voided.
- Rapid administration of IV fluid is contraindicated in children with hypertonic dehydration.
    - RISK = water intoxication resulting in cerebral edema and seizures.
    - Sodium levels in the plasma need to be reduced SLOWLY.
        - Sodium takes more time than water to move in and out of the brain cells.

Oral Rehydration Therapy
- Indicated with:
    - Mild to moderate dehydration

- Rehydration Solution:
  - Pedialyte
- Contraindications:
  - Withholding food or fluids
  - BRAT diet

IV Rehydration
- Indications
  - Severe dehydration
  - Children not tolerating oral rehydration
- Solutions
  - Normal Saline ONLY (Lactated Ringers not recommended by American Academy of Pediatrics)
- Initial Rehydration (Phase I) – ALL types of dehydration
  - 20-30ml/kg IV rapid bolus up to 2-3 times
- Ongoing Rehydration (Phase II)
  - Isotonic and Hypotonic
    - Replace entire fluid and electrolyte deficit in first 24 hours
  - Hypertonic
    - Replace entire fluid and electrolyte deficit in first 48 hours

Case Studies

1. Calculate the hourly and daily maintenance fluid requirements for a child who weighs:
    a. 8 kg

    b. 15 kg

    c. 23 kg

2. Amanda is a 12 month old with gastroenteritis who presents to your ER this afternoon with dehydration. She is irritable with a sunken fontanel and dry mucous membranes. Her mother reports she is not drinking well and has had only 2 wet diapers today. Amanda's HR = 156, RR = 44, BP 80/40. Her serum sodium = is 125. She weighs 9.5 kg.
   a. What is the degree/severity of Amanda's dehydration?

   b. What is the type of dehydration (based on Na level)?

Answers

Case Study #1

a. **hourly**: 8kg X 4ml/hour = <u>32ml/hour</u>

   daily: 8kg X 100ml/day = <u>800ml/day</u>

b. **hourly**: 10kg X 4ml/hour = 40ml/hour + 5kg X 2ml = 10ml/hour = <u>50ml/hour</u>

   daily: 10kg X 100ml/day = 1000ml/day + 5kg X 50ml/day = 250ml/day = <u>1250ml/day</u>

c. **hourly**: 10kg X 4ml/hour = 40ml/hour + 10kg X 2ml/hour = 20ml/hour + 3kc X 1ml/hour = 3ml/hour = <u>63ml/hour</u>

   daily: 10kg X 100ml/kg = 1000ml/day + 10kg X 50ml/kg = 500ml/day + 3kg X 20ml/kg = 60ml/kg = <u>1560ml/day</u>

Case Study #2

a. moderate

b. hypotonic/hyponatremic

Chapter 5: Pediatric Liver Function Tests (LFTs)

Pediatric Liver Function Tests

Pediatric liver function tests (LFTs) are a set of clinical laboratory parameters that are used in primary, acute and critical care nursing of children. It is therefore, important that pediatric nurses understand the LFTs parameters and what deviations from normal values indicate. Many pediatric nurses are overwhelmed and confused by the LFTs and what they mean. Therefore, in this chapter, we will unlock the mystery of the pediatric LFTs interpretation. We will do so by using a pneumonic called *The ABCs of Pediatric LFTs* (Jakubik, Cockerham, Altmann, and Grossman, 2003).

In this chapter we will discuss the following information about pediatric LFTs:
- Anatomy and physiology of the liver
- Liver function tests and their clinical implications
- Comprehensive and organized interpretation of the LFTs using *The ABCs of LFTs* pneumonic

Anatomy and Physiology of the Liver

In order to understand liver function tests it is helpful first to review the anatomy and physiology of the liver. The liver is the largest organ in the body, located in the right upper quadrant under the diaphragm. There are two lobes, right (larger) and left (smaller), separated by the falciform ligament.

Liver Vasculature

The hepatic portal vein receives deoxygenated blood containing nutrients. The hepatic artery receives oxygenated blood. Blood enters the liver and hepatic cells filter oxygen, nutrients, and poisons.

Portal Triad

The portal triad is the hepatic artery, hepatic vein and bile ducts. Hepatocytes secrete bile (800-1000ml/day) which empties into the hepatic ductal system: right and left hepatic ducts (extending from the liver), common hepatic duct, cystic duct (extends from the gallbladder), and common bile duct (excretes bile into the duodenum of the small intestine).

Physiology/Functions of the Liver
The liver has three main functions: vascular, secretory, and metabolic. The vascular function involves the filtration of blood. The secretory function provides for bile synthesis and excretion. The metabolic function involves the metabolism of nutrition and glucose, carbohydrates, proteins and lipids.

Liver Function Tests (LFTs)
The LFTs include the following laboratory tests: bilirubin, enzymes, coagulation studies, and proteins. It is easy to get confused when trying to look at all of the LFTs and what they mean. Therefore, we will use a pneumonic called *The ABCs of LFTs* to help you examine the pediatric LFTs in a comprehensive and organized manner. I have used this method to teach and personally interpret pediatric LFTs for more than a decade and I can assure you that it helps to make LFTs interpretation easy. The remainder of this chapter will take you through *The ABCs of LFTs* pneumonic and will explain how to interpret the LFTs using this pneumonic as a guide.

There are four questions that flow from *The ABCs of LFTs* pneumonic. These questions guide your interpretation of each component of the LFTs. So the first step in using this pneumonic is to memorize the four questions contained within it. Nurse Builders publishes laboratory interpretation prompt cards that can be used as a resource. The bottom line is that the more you use *The ABCs of LFTs* pneumonic, the sooner you will memorize it and have it as a mental resource for interpreting pediatric LFTs. So let's take a look at these four questions.

The ABCs of LFTs
- A: "Ask" 2 questions…
    o Is the bilirubin elevated?
    o Is the liver injured?

- B: B is for "bile" – Is there cholestasis?

- C: "Can" the liver work? (Is the liver working?)

So let's take a look at each component of *The ABCs of LFTs* interpretation.

A: "Ask" Question #1: Is the bilirubin elevated?

Bilirubin
Bilirubin is a byproduct of the breakdown of red blood cells (RBCs) into iron, globin, and bilirubin. It is a bile pigment and is broken down into two types: <u>unconjugated</u> (also called <u>indirect</u>) and <u>conjugated</u> (also called <u>direct</u>).

- <u>Unconjugated (Indirect) Bilirubin</u>
Unconjugated bilirubin is present in the systemic circulation. It is the immediate byproduct of the RBC breakdown and is, therefore, free floating in the systemic circulation. The normal value is 0.2 – 1.0 mg/dl. It is fat soluble and binds to albumin for transport to the liver. It is toxic and, at higher levels, crosses the blood-brain barrier in young infants. However, it does not cross the blood-brain barrier in older infants and children due to their more developed blood-brain barrier. Untreated neonatal hyperbilirubinemia (levels >20-30) can lead to movement disorders and mental retardation, which is a major reason why early

identification and treatment of hyperbilirubinemia in neonates is so important.

Clinical Implications:
<u>Increased unconjugated bilirubin</u> typically indicates RBC turnover (hemolysis) as in neonatal hyperbilirubinemia (physiologic jaundice) and sickle cell disease. It is useful to think of the unconjugated bilirubin as being "before the liver" because unconjugated bilirubin is the type of bilirubin that exists before it has travelled to the liver. An increase in the unconjugated bilirubin, therefore, is usually NOT indicative of liver disease.

- <u>Conjugated (Direct) Bilirubin</u>

Conjugated bilirubin is present in the hepatobiliary system. It is formed when the unconjugated bilirubin enters the liver and is conjugated with glucuronic acid. It is non-toxic, water soluble, and detached from albumin. Its normal value is 0.0 to 0.3 mg/dl. The conjugated bilirubin is excreted into the hepatic ducts, is transported to the intestine, and then is excreted from the body through the stool. The bilirubin is the pigment which gives stool its color.

Clinical Implications:
Increased conjugated bilirubin indicates a build up inside the liver (hepatobiliary system) as in the following conditions: biliary atresia, hepatobiliary obstruction, cholestatic liver disease, and liver synthetic destruction. An increase in the conjugated bilirubin is, therefore, indicative of liver disease.

Helpful Hint: First look at the total bilirubin to evaluate whether or not it is elevated. If the total bilirubin is elevated, next determine whether the unconjugated or conjugated bilirubin is elevated. Elevations in unconjugated bilirubin tell you that the problem is "before the liver" (not liver disease or dysfunction). Elevations in the conjugated bilirubin point to a problem "inside the liver" (liver disease or dysfunction.)

- Total Bilirubin

The normal range for the total bilirubin is 0.2-1.0 mg/dl and is determined by one of the following two formulas:
1. Direct + Indirect
2. Conjugated + Unconjugated + Delta Fraction

The delta fraction is the bilirubin remaining bound to albumin in the systemic circulation (very small amount). It explains the difference between direct (slightly higher) and conjugated bilirubin. In general, it is safe to eliminate the delta fraction in most clinical situations.

> A: "Ask" question #2: Is the liver injured?
> ALT   AST   LDH
>
> ALT, AST, & LDH – Answer question #2: Is the liver injured?

Alanine Aminotransferase (ALT)
The ALT is the most specific enzyme for indicating hepatocellular injury. An <u>increase in ALT</u>, therefore, indicates liver injury. This is because the hepatocytes are the only cells with high amounts of ALT in the body. The normal value for ALT is 10-35 U/L.

Helpful Hint: To remember that elevations in ALT indicate hepatocellular injury, think "L" for liver.

Aspartate Aminotransferase (AST)
AST is present in large amounts in the liver, kidney, RBCs, pancreas, and skeletal muscle.

Therefore, <u>increases in AST</u> will occur with damage to any of these tissues. Normal values for the AST are 15-40 U/L.

Lactic Acid Dehydrogenase (LDH)
LDH is not as specific an indicator for liver function as ALT and AST. It is primarily a cardiac enzyme that is found in the heart, skeletal muscle, brain, kidneys, RBCs, and liver. To assess LDH significance for liver dysfunction ALT and AST need to be elevated. Normal values for LDH are 120-750 U/L.

> **B: B is for "bile"...Is there cholestasis?**
> **GGT ALP**

Cholestasis
Cholestasis is a reduction in the rate of bile flow through the hepatobiliary system. GGT and ALP are the LFTs that indicate cholestasis.

GGT (Gamma Glutamyltransferase)
GGT is present in the liver, bile ducts, small bowel, kidney, brain, pancreas, spleen, and breast. Its normal value is 13-25 U/L. An <u>increase in GGT</u> will be seen with most liver diseases including: hepatobiliary disease, biliary obstruction, and intrahepatic cholestatic

disorders. Elevations can also be seen with alcohol consumption and certain drugs such as anticonvulsants (phenabarbitol and phenytoin) and anticoagulants (warfarin).

ALP (Alkaline Phosphate)
ALP, also called "Alk Phos," is present in the liver, biliary tract, small intestine, bone and kidney. The normal value is 175 – 420 U/L. Elevated ALP can be a normal finding in growing children (especially adolescents). Extreme elevations are present in cholestatic disorders such as intrahepatic and extrahepatic obstructions.

C: "Can" the liver work?
PT/PTT   Ammonia   Albumin

Coagulation Studies
Prothrombin time (PT) and partial thromboplastin time (PTT), the coagulation studies, are predominantly formed in the liver. They reflect coagulation factor activity and liver function at the present time. Increased values (prolonged time) indicate a problem with coagulation activity and, therefore, that the "liver is not working."

- Prothrombin Time (PT)

PT is the laboratory test that measures the time it takes to form a firm clot after tissue thromboplastin (factor III) and calcium are added to a blood sample. Its normal value is 11.5-13.8 seconds. PT measures abnormalities in the extrinsic pathway of the coagulation cascade {factors I (fibrinogen), II (prothrombin), V, VII, and X}. It reflects the synthetic function of the liver if the vitamin K supply is adequate.

- Partial Thromboplastin Time (PTT)

PTT is the laboratory test that measures the time it takes to form a firm clot after phospholipids are added to a blood sample. Its normal value is 26.0 – 38.0 seconds. PTT measures abnormalities in both the intrinsic and common pathways of the coagulation cascade (all coagulation factors except Factor VII). Of these factors, II, IX, & X require vitamin K as a co-factor. Therefore, PTT reflects the synthetic function of the liver if the vitamin K supply is adequate.

Proteins

- Ammonia (NH3)

NH3 is a byproduct of protein breakdown and is largely produced by the colonic bacteria urease. It is converted by the liver into urea, then into glutamine. NH3 is removed during the first hepatic pass of portal blood. Its normal value: 9-33 mm/L. An increase in NH3 may indicate one of the following: GI bleed (due to increased colonic production); increased dietary protein (due to increased colonic production); extrahepatic and intrahepatic shunting of blood; and liver failure.

- Albumin

Albumin is the major circulating protein and is responsible for plasma oncotic pressure. It is totally synthesized in the liver (150mg/kg/day) with a half-life of 21 days. Its normal value: 3.7 – 5.6 gm/dl. A decreased level indicates a chronic rather than an acute problem.

Decreased (hypoalbuminemia) has 2 main causes:
1. Impaired synthetic liver function (i.e. not making it)
    a. Example: liver failure
2. Systemic disease processes that result in losing albumin from the body (i.e. losing it from somewhere)
    a. Examples: protein losing enteropathies and renal disease (nephrotic syndrome)

Case Studies

1. Gabrielle is an 8 day old admitted to your pediatric unit with the following LFTs:
   total bilirubin = 18
   unconjugated bilirubin = 17.2
   conjugated bilirubin = 0.8
   ALT = 22   AST = 27   GGT = 18
   ALP = 202   PT = 12.1   PTT = 30
   NH3 = 17   Albumin = 4.1

   a. What values are abnormal?

   b. What do the abnormalities indicate?

   c. Name a condition consistent with the above LFTs values.

2. Jordan is a 3 month old baby cared for on your pediatric unit after a failed Chasai procedure. His LFTs are as follows:
total bilirubin = 23
unconjugated bilirubin = 1.0
conjugated bilirubin = 22.0
ALT = 89   AST = 76   GGT = 223
ALP = 560   PT = 14.2   PTT = 38
NH3 = 35   Albumin = 4.6

a. What values are abnormal?

b. What do the abnormalities indicate?

c. Name a condition consistent with the above LFTs values.

3. Jason is a 3 year old long-term GI patient who was admitted to your pediatric unit today with a history of a fever with a central line. His LFTs are as follows:
total bilirubin = 26
conjugated bilirubin = 24.3
unconjugated bilirubin = 1.7
ALT = 97   AST = 79   GGT = 249
ALP = 578   PT = 19   PTT = 45
NH3 = 56   Albumin = 2.8

   a. What values are abnormal?

   b. What do the abnormalities indicate?

   c. Name a condition consistent with the above LFTs values.

Answers

Case Study #1
a. Total bilirubin and unconjugated bilirubin are elevated.

b. This indicates that there is a buildup of bilirubin "before the liver" where there is a "traffic jam" getting unconjugated bilirubin into the liver to be conjugated with glucuronic acid.

c. These labs are consistent with neonatal hyperbilirubinemia.

Case Study #2
a. The following values are elevated: total bilirubin, conjugated bilirubin, ALT, AST, GGT, ALP. The PT and PTT are slightly prolonged.

b. This indicated a buildup of conjugated bilirubin "inside the liver" which indicated liver disease. The extreme elevation in GGT and ALP suggest hepatobiliary disease consistent with biliary obstruction.

c. The LFTs listed in combination with the patient's history of a chasai procedure, used for the treatment of biliary atresia, this patient most likely has cholestatic liver disease with hepatobiliary obstruction due to biliary atresia.

Case Study #3
 a. All of Jason's LFTS are elevated.

 b. These elevations are a sign of significant liver disease.

 c. Jason has end stage liver disease and is awaiting a liver transplant.

Chapter 6:
Pediatric Acid-Base Balance

Acid-Base Balance

Acid-base balance involves the regulation of acid in the form of hydrogen ions (H+) in the body fluids in order to promote optimal cell function. Acid-base balance is regulated by the renal, respiratory, and hematologic systems through the regulation of HCO3 (base) and CO2 (acid) to determine serum pH through regulation of hydrogen ions (H+).

Normal Values
The term pH is used to express the H+ concentration of a fluid. Normal pediatric serum pH is 7.35 to 7.45. As the pH fluctuates, the respiratory and renal systems respond in order to regulate H+ ions. The kidneys produce the bicarbonate buffer (HCO3), which acts as a biochemical sponge to soak up excess H+ and also conserves H+ when they are depleted. The lungs remove or conserve carbon dioxide (physiologic acid) by regulating depth and rate of respirations.

Acidosis is defined as a pH of less than 7.35 and reflects either a net loss of HCO3 or gain of CO2. Alkalosis is defined as a pH of greater than 7.45 and reflects either a net gain of HCO3 or loss of CO2.

- The pH system is inversely related to the hydrogen ions:
    - ↑H+ → ↓pH = acidic
    - ↓H+ → ↑pH = alkaline (basic)
- pH = 1 : only H+ ions are present (acid)
- pH = 7 : neutral (distilled water)
- pH = 14 : No H+ ions present (base/alkaline)

Normal pediatric serum HCO3 is 22-26 mEq/L. Normal PaO2 is 80 - 100 mmHg. Normal pediatric PaCO2 is 35 - 45 mmHg. And normal base excess is -2.0 to +2 mEq/L.

Types of Acid-Base Imbalances
- Four types:
    - Respiratory Acidosis
    - Respiratory Alkalosis
    - Metabolic Acidosis
    - Metabolic Alkalosis

Pediatric Laboratory Interpretation | 107

- Interpretation of Acid-Base Imbalances

  Disturbances in acid-base balance can be pulmonary or metabolic in origin. The first step is to look at the pH to determine if it is high or low. Next, look at the CO2 and the HCO3 and determine which is high or low. If the CO2 is abnormal, then the source is respiratory. If the HCO3 is abnormal, then the source is metabolic.
  - <7.35 = acidosis
    - If PaCO2 is >45 = respiratory acidosis
    - If HCO3 is <22 = metabolic acidosis
  - >7.45 = alkalosis
    - If PaCO2 is <35 = respiratory alkalosis
    - If HCO3 is >26 = metabolic alkalosis

- How does regulation work?
  - Normal pediatric serum pH = 7.35-7.45
    - pH < 7.35 = acidosis (net loss of HCO3 or gain of CO2)
    - pH > 7.45 = alkalosis (net gain of HCO3 or loss of CO2)

Memory Jogger: *To remember the direction that pH moves in relation to the CO2 and HCO3 it is helpful to remember the pneumonic ROME. ROME stands for: respiratory opposite, metabolic equal. In respiratory acidosis and alkalosis, the pH and CO2 move in opposite directions, while in metabolic acidosis and alkalosis the pH and HCO3 move in the same direction.*

- "ROME"
  - **R**espiratory **O**pposite
    - pH ↓ CO2 ↑
    - pH ↑ CO2 ↓
  - **M**etabolic **E**qual
    - pH ↓ HCO3 ↓
    - pH ↑ HCO3 ↑

So let's take a closer look at each type of acid-base imbalance and what causes them.

- <u>Respiratory Acidosis</u>

Respiratory acidosis occurs because of an excess in CO2. Increases in blood CO2 levels, decrease blood pH and create surplus carbonic acid. Causes of respiratory acidosis are: hypoventilation, respiratory arrest, COPD, and CNS depression. Treatment is geared at increasing the respiratory rate to blow off CO_2 and may include 100% oxygen via face mask.

- Respiratory Alkalosis

Respiratory alkalosis occurs when there is a CO_2 deficit. Decreased CO_2 levels and increased blood pH, results in lowered carbonic acid blood levels. Causes of respiratory alkalosis are hyperventilation, which occurs during fear, anxiety, and pulmonary infections. Signs and symptoms of respiratory alkalosis include: hyperventilation, numbness, prickling or tingling, altered level of consciousness, agitation, and even unresponsiveness. Treatment is geared to controlling the respiratory rate, calming the patient, and having the child breathe into a non-rebreather mask with reduced oxygen flow.

- Metabolic Acidosis

Metabolic acidosis occurs when bicarbonate levels are low in relation to carbonic acid levels. The kidneys fail to produce sufficient bicarbonate in response to decreased blood pH levels. The most common cause of metabolic acidosis in kids is prolonged or severe diarrhea which causes loss of HCO_3 in the stool. Other causes include renal impairment and diabetic ketoacidosis. Signs and symptoms include: kussmaul breathing, weakness, disorientation, and even coma. Treatment is aimed at reducing CO_2 levels through hyperventilation and administering bicarbonate in severe cases.

- Metabolic Alkalosis

Metabolic alkalosis occurs when bicarbonate levels are too high. This typically occurs when the body loses chloride and hydrogen ions. The most common cause in children is prolonged vomiting. Signs and symptoms include slow, shallow respirations (compensation) and altered level of consciousness. The treatment is to address the underlying cause.

Case Studies

1. The child you are caring for has the following lab results:
   pH = 7.28 CO_2 = 50 HCO_3 = 24
   a. What acid-base imbalance does your patient have?

2. The child you are caring for has the following lab results:
   a. What acid-base imbalance does your patient have?
   pH = 7.26 CO_2 = 40 HCO_3 = 19

3. The child you are caring for has the following lab results:
   a. What acid-base imbalance does your patient have?
   pH = 7.49 CO_2 = 32 HCO_3 = 25

4. The child you are caring for has the following lab results:
   a. What acid-base imbalance does your patient have?
   pH = 7.51 CO_2 = 38 HCO_3 = 29

Answers

Case Study #1
   a. Respiratory acidosis – the pH is < 7.35 and the CO2 is elevated with a normal HCO3.

Case Study #2
   a. Metabolic acidosis – the pH is < 7.35 and the HCO3 is low with a normal CO2.

Case Study #3
   a. Respiratory alkalosis – the pH is > 7.45 and the CO2 is low with a normal HCO3.

Case Study #4
   a. Metabolic acidosis – the pH is > 7.45 and the HCO3 is elevated with a normal CO2.

Reference List

Corbett, J. V. (2000). *Laboratory Tests and Diagnostic Procedures with Nursing Diagnosis (5th ed.)* Upper Saddle River, New Jersey: Prentice Hall Health.

Guyton, A. C. & Hall, J. E. (2000). *Textbook of Medical Physiology (3rd ed.).* Philadelphia: W. B. Saunders Company.

Jakubik, L. D., Cockerham, J., Altmann, A., & Grossman, M. B. (2003). The ABCs of pediatric laboratory interpretation: Understanding the CBC with differential and LFTs. *Pediatric Nursing, 29*(2), 97-103.

Kee, J. L. (1999). *Laboratory and Diagnostic Test with Nursing Implications (5th ed.).* Stamford, Connecticut: Appleton and Lange.

Malarkey, L.M. & McMorrow, M. E. (Eds.) (2000). *Nurse's Manual of Laboratory Tests and Diagnostic Procedures* (2nd ed.). Philadelphia: W. B. Saunders Company.

Muscari, M. E. (2004). Lippincott's Review Series: Pediatric Nursing (4th ed.). Philadelphia: Lippincott Williams & Wilkins.

Made in the USA
Charleston, SC
22 August 2013